Get Fit On The Go

75 Intense Workouts To Keep You In Shape On The Road

Introduction

I want to thank you and congratulate you for downloading the book, "How To Deal With Death: The Comprehensive Guide to Overcoming Your Emotional Stress."

This book contains proven steps and strategies on how to stay in shape away from home.

Most of us workout as often as we need to and without any restrictions, but sometimes life gets in the way and you're not able to make it to the gym or you just flat out don't want to. That's okay. Whether you're working late to beat a deadline or you're travelling, don't worry one bit. There are ways to balance work, home life, and fitness – especially on the road.

If you're one of the many people who often go on business trips or any work related travel, chances are that you might need to skip some of your normal routine. When you're travelling, you'll most likely face some of the common scenarios below:

No access to a gym – working out in a gym is usually the most ideal place since it has most of the top equipment around. However, when you're on a business trip, you can't always expect to have enough time to go to a gym or perhaps there isn't one to go to at all. Most hotels have fitness centers but these "fitness centers" might have about three to five small machines and a couple of treadmills. Certainly less than ideal.

Limited types of meals – One of the most difficult things to do when on the road is sticking with your diet. You won't have any access to the normal things you have at home like a fridge or a kitchen and chances are you won't be able to prepare healthy meals to complete your diet.

<u>Odd sleeping hours</u> – Though this may only apply if you're going to cross different time zones but it does happen a lot. It's tough to get a good night's sleep if you came from one time zone to another. Although it takes just a few days to set your body clock to normal again it sure is tough to go through the adjustment period.

<u>Pressure, pressure, pressure!</u> – This mostly happens if in any case you're travelling on a business trip that requires you to go the extra mile. In any other case, the mere fact that you're out of your comfort zone is pressure enough.

<u>Unfamiliar surroundings</u> – although researching beforehand sort of compensates for the new surroundings but it just doesn't feel like home. It's hard to get around a place that you barely know of.

<u>The unexpected becomes the expected</u> – basically a lot of things could happen when you're on a trip. You may forgot a thing or two in your baggage or perhaps you forgot a couple of details in your game plan. Things happen and the sad part is you can't always predict what's going to transpire next.

Thanks again for downloading this book, I hope you enjoy it!

Travel Workout Essentials

Here are a couple of ideas that will help you figure out a way to buy some time to work out while travelling:

Plan ahead of time – planning is always essential when travelling. If you're going to be leaving for a business trip, you'll find it very useful to plan everything ahead. It helps a lot to list down the things that you are going to be doing on your trip. Jot down some notes or perhaps create a list of your schedules on your smartphone or computer. Anticipate every single thing that might happen and create backup plans if anything goes out of order. Listing the things you'll do on your trip beforehand will make it easier for you to allocate some of your time to hit the gym at your destination. If you're traveling through different time zones, beat the jet lag by pushing yourself until it's time for you to go to bed. Don't doze off just yet when you reach your room. There's plenty of time to rest when it's time for bed. This will set your body clock to the appropriate time zone. Also, don't skip meals nor indulge yourself with delightful midnight snacks. Although it satisfies the craving but it does nothing good for you than gaining unhealthy weight.

Pack the right stuff – traveling surely denies us of access to things that we usually use especially for working out. But do you really need to be bound by these restrictions? Of course not! The trick here is to pack the right stuff. Bring along the stuff that you'll find pretty useful like sneakers, workout clothes, and headphones.

Pick the right place – this may not apply to all trips as some might have a specified location prepared for you to stay. In cases where you can choose the hotel you're going to be staying in, check to see if it has a gym. Some companies may reimburse the gym fees acquired during business trips. It helps to double check if your company will compensate for those kind of expenses just to make sure that you won't be spending your own. Most of the time this isn't much of the case. When it comes to maintaining a fit and healthy body, all you need is a little bit of creativity and persistence. All you need to do is make use of what's available at hand. Take the stairs instead of the elevator; It's an alternative cardio exercise and it's pretty effective and pretty much works in any establishment that has stairs. Walk as often as you can. It can actually let you burn a lot of calories keeping you fit and lose weight at the same time.

Find an alternative and be creative – if you're out of luck with your hotel not having a gym or a fitness center nearby, it's best to find an alternative way to workout. Basically, the difference between working out in a gym and in a hotel room is the equipment. Body weight workouts are your best option to keep your body in shape without leaving your hotel room. It's useful to be familiar with how to properly do push-ups, squats, lunges, and other body weight exercises. If you're used to going on a morning jog, do it! Just remember to be careful if you're in a place that you're not familiar with. If all else fails and you don't seem to have any option left, you could always use an empty parking lot to jog or perhaps the sidewalks near your hotel. If you're thinking this is way over for you, don't! Fit people usually aren't the timid ones. Pack along a resistance band just in case. Its light, you wouldn't even notice that it's there but it works! Another thing you would want to consider is Yoga. With Yoga, all you need is your trusty Yoga mat and you're ready to complete one whole session to keep you fit the rest of your journey.

Make food your priority – traveling is both time consuming and taxing on the body. You'll need all the nutrients you can get out of food and be sure to get plenty of them. Always bear in mind that you need to gain healthy weight while on your trip. This will let you keep up with your busy schedule without wearing out. Other than filing up with nutritious food, make it a habit to constantly rehydrate. Water does a great deal of help in keeping you from being easily tired. Just because you ate something that doesn't mean it's healthy for you nor will it suffice your body's needs. Bear in mind that each person has different needs than others. Some may require specific food, different vitamins and minerals, and amounts unlike others. Be sure to get what you need every single time and do not forget to enjoy your every meal.

Commit to being fit – after a long journey it's very tempting to hit the sack and relax. However, you must commit yourself to working out every single day of your travel even at least an hour. After all, the most challenging bit isn't the lack of a fitness center or a gym. It's the lack of commitment to workout that's the most challenging thing to conquer. No matter what your schedule would be, be sure to pack a lot of commitment with you. It's the number one thing you're going to need to work out while travelling. It's normal to want to think of relaxing or going out for the night but think about your priorities. However, things are quite different when you're away from home and you need to have a little more discipline.

Be comfortable – sometimes the first time that we encounter changes in our routine we tend to hate it. Not to say that everyone hates changes but it's rather common to find it hard to do something else rather than what you're used to. If you're pretty used to using gym equipment, better make yourself comfortable working out without them. If you're traveling it's likely that you'll end up in some place where gym equipment isn't available. The trick is to be comfortable at what you're doing. Don't be bothered by the fact that you might need to improvise, be proud of it! The success stories you usually read about on the Internet aren't based on timid people. It's about those who show they can think beyond the box and actually achieve their goals because they were comfortable with what they're doing.

Set your goals straight – other than being prepared and committed, you must also set goals for yourself. Just like your normal routine to the gym several times a week, knowing what you need to accomplish for the rest of your trip is important. This will give you enough time for everything. Let's say you're traveling on a business trip and every minute counts, how do you plan on managing your time? It's a matter of goals, priorities, and of course, simple math. Remember that aside from your trip, you have your fitness as a part of the list of your top priorities. Take some time to develop a scheme on what workout routines you want to accomplish each day. Set a goal that's balanced. Something that's not too hard and does not consume a huge portion of your time.

Find the perfect workout – one thing that you should always keep in mind is looking for the best travel workout. Working out comes in many forms. Some variations may require equipment like the ones they teach you at the gym while others can be completed by harnessing bodyweight. It's important to understand what type of workout you need to do when you're travelling. This will allow you to squeeze in the perfect workouts for the little time you have after everything else has been done. Since most of the travel workouts involve using your bodyweight instead of gym equipment, it won't be as intensive but as equally effective.

75 No-Equipment Body Weight Work out Routines

Here are 75 high-intensity workouts. Some of you cross fitters may recognize them. Many of these come from the best trainers around the world. You won't need any gym equipment. At the most you'll need a jump rope and a pavement to do your runs. If you don't like running in an unfamiliar city, try running sprints in the hotel parking lot – just a thought.

Don't cheat yourself! Give it your all. Before you start working out, ensure that you're properly warming up and stretching!

1.

Sprint 100 meters

Rest 1 minute

Repeat 10 times

2.

100 Single under (Jump Rope)

50 Squats

5 rounds for time

3.

AMRAP in 20 minutes:

-10 Burpees

-15 Squats

-20 Knees-to-chin (laying down)

4.

10 Rounds of:

-10 Broad Jump Burpees

-10 Jumping Lunges

5.

10 rounds of

- 10 burpees

- 10 sit-ups

6.

5 Rounds

-15m Bear Crawl

-20 Push-ups

-15m Crab Walk

-20 Jump Squats

-15m Broad Jump Burpees

-20 Mountain Climbers

7.

3 rounds for time

-Run 1/2 mile

-50 squats

8.

10 Rounds for time

-10 push-ups

-10 sit ups

-10 squats

9.

200 squats for time

10.

5 rounds for time

- Run 200m

- 10 squats

- 10 push-ups

11.

3 rounds for time

- Sprint 200m

- 25-push ups

12.

Tabata Squats and Push-ups:

20 seconds on 10 seconds rest, 8 rounds each.

Count your lowest score.

13.

20 rounds for time

- 5 push-ups

- - 5 squats

- 5 sit ups

14.

Invisible Fran:

21-15-9 for time

-Squats

-Push-ups

15.

6 rounds for time

- 10 push-ups

- 10 squats

- 10 sit ups

16.

5 rounds for time

- 25 Single sit ups

- 50 Squats

17.

Pushups

Sit-ups

50-40-30-20-10 Rep Rounds for Time

18.

5 Rounds for Time

- 3 vertical jumps

- 3 squats

- 3 long jumps

19.

100 Squats for Time

20.

10 Rounds for Time

- 10 Push-ups

- 10 Squats

- 10 Sit-ups

21.

10-9-8-7-6-5-4-3-2-1

- Burpees

- Sit ups

22.

5 Rounds for Time

- Run 400 meters (1:30-2:30 minutes)

- 30 Squats

23.

250 jumping jacks For Time

24.

5 Rounds – Count Squats

- Run 1 minute

- Squat for 1 minute

25.

Run 1 mile and do 10 push-ups every 1 minute.

26.

Handstand practice, 25 tries at free handstands, then a 1 mile run

27.

10 Rounds for Time

- 10 push-ups

- 10 squats

28.

For Time

- 100 jumping jacks

- 75 squats

- 50 push ups

- 25 burpees

29.

100 Push-ups for Time

30.

5 Rounds for Time

- 10 vertical jumps

- run 400m

31.

10 Rounds for Time

- 10 Push-ups

- 100m Sprint

32.

5 Rounds for Time

- Handstand 30 seconds

- 20 squats

33.

4 Rounds for Time

- 10 vertical jumps

- 10 push-ups

- 10 sit ups

34.

- 2 minute max push ups

- 1 minute break

- 2 minutes max sit ups

- 1 minute break

- 2 minute max squats

35.

5 Rounds for Time

- 20 Lunge steps

- 20 squats

- 10 pushups

36.

100 Burpees for Time

37.

7 Rounds for Time

- 7 Squats

- 7 Burpees

38.

10 Rounds for Time

- Sprint 100m

- Walk 100m

39.

3 Rounds for Time

- 50 sit-ups

- 400m run walk

40.

10 Rounds for Time

- 10 walking lunges

- 10 push-ups

41.

10 Rounds for Time

- 10 burpees

- 100meter sprint

42.

4 Rounds for Time

- Run 400m

- 50 squats

43.

Run 1 mile and do 10 push-ups every 1 minute.

44.

5 Rounds for Time

- Ten vertical jumps (jump as high as you can, land and do it again)

- 10 push-ups

45.

3 Rounds for Time

- 20 jumping jacks

- 20 burpees

- 20 squats

46.

5 Rounds for Time

-30 second handstand against a wall,

- Followed by a 30 second static hold at the bottom of the squat

47.

Run 1 mile for time.

48.

3 Rounds for Time

- Run 200m

- 50 squats

49.

25 reps for time

- Handstand 10 seconds jack-knife to vertical jump

50.

50-40-30-20-10 Rep Rounds for Time

- Single under (Jump Rope)

- Pushups

51.

AMRAP in 10 minutes

- 3 Burpees

- 4 pushups

- 5 squats

52.

10 rounds

- 30 second squat jump

- 30 second rest

53.

4 rounds for time

- 1/2 mile run

- 50 squats

54.

3 Rounds for Time

- 20 tuck jumps

- 30 second handstands

55.

8 Rounds for Time

- Sprint 100m

- 30 squats

56.

Sprint for 30 seconds, do 20 pushups

--30 second rest—

Repeat 5x

57.

20 Rounds for Time

- 5 squats

- 5 push-ups

- 5 sit ups

58.

For Time

Run 1 mile with 100 squats at midpoint

59.

10 Rounds for Time

- 10 sit ups

- 10 burpees

60.

Bottom to bottom squats

8 Rounds

20 second of work and 10 seconds of a squat hold

Run 1 mile

61.

10 Rounds

- Handstand hold, 30 seconds,

- Squat hold 30 seconds

62.

4 Rounds for Time

- 20 sit ups

- 20 push-ups

- 400m Run

63.

100 squats

3 min. rest

100 squats

64.

3 Rounds for Time

- Run 200m

- 50 squats

65.

5 Rounds for Time

- With eyes closed do 10 squats with open eyes

- Do 10 pushups eyes closed

66.

10 Rounds for Time

- Run 100m

- 20 squats

67.

Test yourself on a max set of pushups, tight body chest to the floor, full extension!

68.

Tabata Tuck jumps and Sit-ups:

20 seconds on 10 seconds rest, 8 rounds each.

Count your lowest score.

69.

Run 1 mile, stopping every minute to do 20 squats.

70.

3 Rounds for Time

- 20 Squats

- 20 Burpees

- 20 Push-Ups

71.

For Time

- 25 squats

- 5 push-ups

- 20 squat

- 10 push-ups

- 15 squat

- 15 push-ups

- 10 squat

- 20 push-ups

- 5 squat

- 25 push-ups

72.

5 Rounds for Time

- 50 Step-ups or Box Jumps

- 10 Burpees

73.

Tabata Squats with eyes closed:

20 seconds on 10 seconds rest, 8 rounds.

Count your lowest score

74.

4 Rounds for Time

- 50 squats

Rest for 2 minutes between rounds.

75.

5 Rounds for Time

- 20 Lunge Steps

- 20 Squats

- 10 Push-ups

Keep Track and Plan Ahead

Going on a trip usually brings about changes in our routine especially when it comes to working out. However, do you really need to skip your workouts just to have more time for your trip? Be informed, be focused, and let your goal be your driving force! There's a lot more that you can do and achieve if you're well informed. Pair it with the right mindset and you're going to be fit no matter where you go, how long you'll stay, and how busy your schedule may be!

Conclusion

Thank you again for downloading this book!

I hope this book was able to help you to achieve or maintain your fitness goals while traveling.

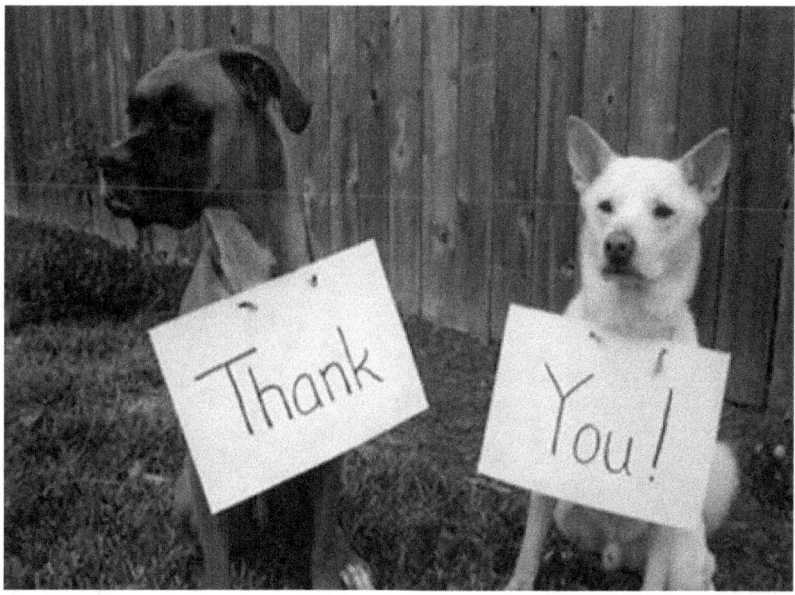

Finally, if you enjoyed this book, then I'd like to ask you for a favor, would you be kind enough to leave a review for this book on Amazon? It'd be greatly appreciated!

Thank you and good luck!

www.ingramcontent.com/pod-product-compliance
Lightning Source LLC
Chambersburg PA
CBHW070527290526
45790CB00003B/1332